MAN WITHOUT

WITHOUT

PORN

GUIDE TO LIVING A

PORN

Steven B. Romero

CONTENT

Sexualizing society

The word "sexualization" refers to the increase of sexually explicit allusions in Western societies since the turn of the twenty-first century in a variety of media and popular culture. As a result of the prevalence of themes from pornography in modern Western media, some have dubbed this cultural change "porno chic" or "raunch culture" (McNair, 2002). (Levy, 2005). The extent to which these changes can be seen as a form of liberation (especially for women) from the oppressive regulation of respectable sexuality is the subject of current debates about sexualization. On the other hand, there is the argument that these representations fail to address the underlying sexism in these cultures and merely offer new ways to regulate and discipline (especially women's) sexuality

Both media representational techniques and the everyday material behaviors of both men and women are considered to be a part of sexualization. the specification of culture.

How many movies have you seen when a high school girl attends a frat party disguised as a college student? Imagine a television scenario where a youngster is made fun of for not having sexual activity yet. Pornography is particularly problematic in this regard; millions of movies exist in which an actress who is eighteen years old is done up to seem much younger, instilling the notion that engaging in sexual activity with girls as young as fourteen is acceptable and normal.

Porn's effects on relationships

How frequently has a character in a TV show or movie expressed astonishment that another one didn't lose their virginity when they were still teenagers? How many times have you seen older guys making advances toward much younger ladies in fictional media? How often have you seen characters who are purported to be young females but who may easily be 25 years old?

Teenagers being sexualized in our media has long been an issue, but we are just now beginning to understand the harm it does. Continue reading to find out more about the effects of early sexualization and how to combat it.With the recent release of the film 50 Shades of Grey, our society has once again addressed significant sexual concerns that are often not discussed or explained to the point where we can learn lessons that can truly enhance our relationships. I will thus use this chance to discuss how pornography impacts the emotional closeness in romantic relationships. I'll begin with a query that I just received.

My spouse has been surreptitiously watching pornographic content online for years, and I only just learned about it. This finding offends me, and the idea of what he's seeing makes me feel disgusting. He doesn't think it's a big problem since I informed him about it. "All males use porn," he asserts. I need a dose of realism. Is male pornography so common? What should I do with these emotions, then?

Many couples have trouble figuring out this crucial issue. In the first place, indeed, a lot of males regularly watch porn. An estimated 40 million Americans frequently use pornographic websites. However, it's not just guys. Women make up around one-third of those frequent visitors. However, it is incorrect to say that pornography is not a "huge concern."

Because it destroys the physical and emotional closeness in genuine relationships, it is a major matter.

Here are a few things to think about:

Trust is the foundation of happy partnerships. Being intimate with someone puts you in a vulnerable position. Trust is the confidence that your spouse will honor you and appreciate your vulnerabilities. It betrays your trust when your spouse discreetly invites others—strangers, no less—into the private space that should be kept for the two of you, and emotions of violation often follow. It takes time and effort to mend a broken trust.

The capacity of the pair to develop emotional connection is the cornerstone to a solid, sustainable relationship. Relationships are more significant when there is emotional, not sexual, connection. Of course, if you take your cues from porn sites or even the constant messages being broadcast by the media, you could believe that sex is the main force that holds partnerships together. Although this misconception is widespread in our sex-obsessed society, emotional connection is what creates feelings of worth, esteem, love, caring, and appreciation in others. Two persons are far more likely to be satisfied with their sexual union when there is emotional connection between them. There is no need to seek out other sources of sexual pleasure or amusement outside of that connection.

Pornography instills irrational expectations in you about your partner and their sexual propensities. Because it gives people a completely erroneous idea of what a normal body looks like and what sexual action is really about, pornography has been found to undermine commitment in relationships. The sexual connection is designed to be a fulfilling way for both partners to show their love for one another. Porn, on the other hand, focuses on self-gratification and often entails controlling or abusing the other person.

I've discovered that folks who had love deficiencies early in life are more likely to use pornography. They often came from households where affection and love were in little supply. We're all ultimately exposed to porn, but those who are lacking in affection tend to be more attracted to it as a replacement for the loving connections they lacked in real life. It may develop into a compulsive activity that might eventually develop into an addiction if the individual often returns to porn to acquire that sensation. Keep fighting to drive these individuals from your bedroom and imagination. Your marriage could be on the line.

Where Sexualization Takes Place

sexualization is so pervasive in our culture, we often fail to recognize it when it is in front of us. It's possible to begin to impress that sexuality by attending an event like a pageant where young girls are dressed in provocative attire. And you don't have to go far in the media to see that young people are being oversexualized on a massive scale.

How many movies have you seen when a high school girl attends a frat party disguised as a college student? Imagine a television scenario where a youngster is made fun of for not having sexual activity yet. Pornography is particularly problematic in this regard; millions of movies exist in which an actress who is eighteen years old is done up to seem much younger, instilling the notion that engaging in sexual activity with girls as young as fourteen is acceptable and normal.

Even female superheroes often dress provocatively and move indecently. In fact, we find it silly when the roles are reversed since feminine characters move so differently from male ones.

Additionally, you'll note that female armor includes a variety of "strategic" cuts if you've ever compared male and female armor in an action video game.

How early the GHoversexualization of young people starts would surprise you. For instance, how many times have you heard someone refer to your young son as a "stud" if you have children? How many people have mentioned your infant girl is already shattering hearts after seeing her?

When the youngster is old enough to comprehend some of the messages, it still continues. Preschooler sizes of thongs with the phrases "Eye Candy" and "Wink Wink" are available. Dolls are shown wearing things like crop tops, short skirts, and fishnet stockings.

What Makes Girls Targets

We've been concentrating on media that sexualizes young girls, as you may have observed. This isn't because boys aren't targets; in fact, we'll talk more about the negative effects of this sexualization on boys later. However, females are often the victims of overt sexualization and the violence that results from it.

The fact that females are targeted so much more often than boys has a cyclical component. Our culture promotes the idea that women are only elevated sex objects. This prompts companies of toys, clothes, video games, advertisements, and everything else to produce more goods based on this stereotype, which furthers the specification of children.

Effects of Negative Gender Stereotypes

Numerous harmful gender stereotypes have their roots in this sexualization. Girls and women are stereotypically represented as being sexually open to males and obedient to them. As we'll see in a minute, these preconceptions may harm relationships between men and women as well as lead to violence. Men are supposed to be the stoic guardians. Children turn to the media and the people in their environment for examples of how to behave. They believe it is the

normal way to behave and interact when
they observe such hypersexual
stereotypes. And as kids become older,
everything around them keeps sending
them these signals.

The Role of Stereotypes in Violence

One in four women encounter intimate
partner violence, one in six women
experience sexual assault, and more than
1.5 million women were victims of violent
crime every year, all of which may be
attributed in large part to gender
stereotypes. Because they are persuaded
that their position is one of subservience,
women think that violence against
intimate partners is normal and
acceptable. They are informed that their
sexuality is the only thing that makes
them valuable.
Men are taught to see women as a
commodity to be enjoyed by them.
Because they have earned the right to
women's attention as men, getting their
consent is not necessary. Men are
perplexed and incensed when women
don't follow this passive sexuality
because they feel cheated out of
something they have a right to.

Issues with Sexualization and Body Image

Women have irrational expectations
about how their bodies should seem as a
result of this hyper-sexualization. Tiny
waistlines, large busts, and rounded hips
are all physical proportions that women
in television and film struggle mightily to
accomplish. And these characters talk a
lot about how they want to lose weight,
how their bodies are what attract guys,
and how men are the center of their
existence.
Things only become worse when you
start playing video games and buying
toys. Designers may construct ladies
whose ideal of beauty is practically
unattainable because they are not
constrained by the limitations of reality.
Women and girls learn to only notice the
ways their bodies fall short when they are
exposed to all of these unattainable role
models.

Issues with body image and health

If you don't think that body image
concerns are a major matter, you should
realize that an eating disorder claims the
life of another person every hour. In the
United States, at least 30 million
individuals struggle with an eating
problem. The mortality rate for eating

disorders is higher than for any other mental condition, including depression.

Even without eating disorders, women and girls could feel pressured to do very risky actions to meet the unattainable beauty standards they see in the media. The least of these concerns is the Kylie Jenner problem. Women who experience self-loathing for falling short in this one crucial area may resort to risky fad diets, painful and costly cosmetic surgery, or even drug misuse as a coping mechanism.

Effects on Teenage Boys

As we've already discussed, this hypersexualization affects people of all ages. Boys learn at a young age that their roles are those of the promiscuous stud and the stern guardian. They are urged to suppress their feelings, "take things like a man," and find women as often as they can.

Men may lash out violently toward women as a result of the repressed wrath brought on by this toxic masculinity culture. Boys could experience peer pressure to begin sexual experimentation before they're ready. When they contrast themselves with superheroes who have the body types of Doritos and early Captain America, males too struggle with body image concerns.

The forces we've spoken about thus far have all existed for many years and in some instances even centuries. Social media, however, has emerged as a new player in the past ten to fifteen years. Today's youth see impossibly high expectations every waking minute of the day, and they come from peers in their eyes.

Teenagers may feel under pressure to live up to an unattainable ideal that Instagram models present. Photoshopping, filters, and angles may work wonders, yet the photographs are presented as truth. Additionally, teenagers are using social media at earlier and younger ages, and they are beginning to take in those harmful messages. Only one possibly internet-related addiction is now acknowledged by the American Psychiatric Association (APA), and that is online gaming. The Diagnostic and Statistical Manual of Mental Disorders, Fifth Edition does not include pornography addiction as a subtype of hypersexual disorder, despite APA consideration. However, online pornography addictions may contain a comparable structure and fundamental principles to drug addiction, according to a neuroscientific study.

Pornography is now so widely accessible thanks to the Internet that avoiding it has become nearly as challenging. As couples try to find a mutually beneficial absorption (or exile) of porn, research is increasingly demonstrating the detrimental effects that pornography is having on relationships. We also know that porn is becoming a significant issue for kids and teens. Research has consistently shown that kids are using the Internet to obtain pornography at younger and younger ages. According to research that was published in the journal Paediatrics, 42 percent of kids and teens between the ages of 10 and 17 have reportedly seen porn. Such early introduction to pornography, which may be quite explicit and gruesome, can cause it to become ingrained in people's daily life.

So, as we get closer to World Mental Health Day on October 10, we must assess the influence that pornography has on our mental health as well as its place in our daily lives and that of our families.

According to a recent study, our mental health may be impacted by pornography in addition to other factors, which was published in September in the journal Psychology of Addictive Behaviors. Instead, research seems that how we view our usage of pornography is related to how we think and feel poorly about ourselves. Depression, rage, and anxiety are particularly linked to internet pornography addiction. The experts contend that what causes mental health suffering is our addictive nature and sensation of being in control.

Porn addictions are similar to other addictions in that individuals seek out porn (as they would drug) because they have acquired a psychological demand rather than because they find it enjoyable, according to researchers in Cambridge, UK.

Frequent exposure to porn creates a form of tolerance where more severe, uncommon, explicit, or deviant sexual pictures and movies are needed to get the same "buzz." Pornography "nearly lodges itself into your consciousness, like a parasite draining away the rest of your life," according to a user who participated in a 2007 research.

Even when our use of pornography is casual, irregular, and rare rather than compulsive, we might nevertheless experience a great deal of stress as a result of it. The interaction between pornography and our relationships is the main source of stress. A lot of couples are attempting to figure out how to handle porn in their relationships. Some couples claim to have used porn to improve their sex life. Others want to avoid using it at all costs. And a third group is finding that there is disagreement among them regarding the use of
porn. Pornography viewing is typically done alone for sexual gratification. We should truly consider how this will affect how we feel about our partners, how we

see them, and if it would be positive or negative for our relationship.

This is especially true when we take into account the power dynamic—or, more accurately, the imbalance—between those participating in the pornographic content we watch. How does our perception of how relationships ought to work change depending on the degree of consent or amount of aggressiveness that is expressed or inferred in porn? Even the sexual actions themselves will have an impact on us because of how detailed they are. Our expectations will also be shaped by the visible body image signals (the size of breasts, waists, bottoms, musculature, or penises that appear to be attractive), which may also play into our fears.

Even when partners are unable to come to terms with their individual or joint use of pornography, it is still preferable that they at least acknowledge the likelihood that at least one of their lives includes pornography.

Situations in which pornography is secretly influencing mood, desire, and libido are far more harmful.

There are several tales of women (usually) who feel justifiably cheated and duped by their husbands' behavior when the husband has been a clandestine user of pornography. One research detailed how women who learned their boyfriend was using pornography felt sexually unappealing and considered the behavior humiliating.

Therefore, whether you are an adult who has to assess your own, or your partner's, use of porn, or whether you are a parent who needs to consider how (and when) pornography will start to impact your child's perception of the world, it will be a live problem that probably touches us all. Consider how pornography may or may not be affecting your mood, your relationships, and your life in light of the upcoming World Mental Health Day.

Porn and depression: a connection

AASECT asserts that individuals may suffer detrimental physical, spiritual, or psychological effects as a result of their sexual urges, thoughts, or actions, such as viewing pornographic material. However, the theory that viewing pornography can cause depression is not currently supported by enough evidence. Despite this, research has discovered some connections between the two.

One 2019 study, for instance, which polled 507 women and 250 men, discovered that depression appeared to increase the risk of having a problematic relationship with pornography. However, this was only true for those who turned to pornography to block out negative feelings. women who use pornography and have sexual issues. According to 2019 research, both men and women who watch too much pornographic content are at an elevated risk of developing depression.

The frequency and duration of a person's exposure to pornography seem to influence the likelihood that they would suffer depression concurrently with or as a result of that usage.

For instance, a 2017 research that polled 582 senior male students found that 14.6 percent of those who admitted accessing pornography more than three times per week reported suffering depression, compared to 2.8 percent of those who said they used it less often.

The same research discovered that the rates of depression were 11.7 percent, 7.1 percent, 4.9 percent, and 5.9 percent, respectively, among those who began using pornography in elementary school, junior middle school, high school, or university. People who morally disapprove of pornography may also be more like to regard their connection with porn as addiction and to experience sexual shame, both of which may increase depression levels. Additionally, problematic pornographic usage seems to be associated with:

- loneliness\sanxiety\sheadaches
- narcissism
- neuroticism
- decreased contentment with life, love, and relationships

Can depression result in using pornography?   There isn't enough solid data to say that sadness may cause a person to get addicted to pornography.

Pornography addiction isn't recognized as a mental health disease by the AASECT.

When compulsive pornographic users' brains were examined after exposure to sexual pictures, it was discovered that their brain activity patterns matched those of patients with alcohol use disorders who viewed alcohol ads. Other studies, however, seem to indicate that this is not the case.

Additionally, several early and small-scale research has revealed that individuals, particularly males, may watch more porn while depressed.

For instance, a 2017 research indicated that males with depression, particularly those who morally oppose pornography, may use it more often as a coping mechanism.

Additionally, a forthcoming research contends that returning male U.S. soldiers with depression are more likely to acquire problematic pornographic usage. Additionally, some studies imply that sadness may alter how someone's usage of pornography is seen or perceived adversely.

According to a 2018 research, melancholy and loneliness were the underlying factors that impacted how online behaviors like viewing pornography affected life satisfaction.

Pornographic triggers

"If you know the opponent and know yourself, you need not dread the conclusion of a hundred wars," the great military thinker Sun Tzu reportedly observed. Knowing your triggers and the stimuli around you is essential to winning the war against porn.

The term "HALT" is often used by therapists to refer to the four states—hunger, anger, loneliness, and tiredness—that might act as triggers for addictive behavior. When pondering your triggers, this is a wonderful place to start. However, everyone is unique, and this is particularly true when it comes to triggers for porn.

Every potential cause is tough to pin down. The three main kinds of porn triggers—environmental, bodily, and emotional—might be useful to consider. We'll look at some of the many ways that these triggers might appear and some doable countermeasures.

1. Environment-related factors
Pornographic material is all around us. Our culture is very sexualized. The sexualization of entertainment and advertising is extreme. The internet is many of places where you may find porn. It might be challenging to stay away from triggers that can threaten to take you off the road to recovery in sexualized surroundings.

Situational awareness—knowing where you're going and what you're going to face—is required in response to environmental stimuli. It's crucial to keep in mind that certain locations are more prone to provoke anxiety than others. At the beach, you're more likely to encounter sexual temptation than at church. The mall is more likely to include triggering visuals than the post office. Michael Johnson describes a disturbing website he visited:

"I was searching through the game schedule on the Tennessee Titans website when I came upon The Cheerleader Button. That's not porn, I overheard someone remark on one side. There won't be any nude people. Everyone will be dressed to the hilt [roughly speaking, of course]. There won't be anything you'll need to admit afterwards.'

Do you often go somewhere that sets you off?

Do you watch any movies or TV programs that make you feel triggered?

Do any webpages make you feel triggered?

The cheerleading button could be to blame. It may be a sexual moment in a movie you like, or it could be Victoria's Secret advertising you see at the mall. What triggering factors in the surroundings might make you turn to porn?

Strategies for Redirecting Environmental Triggers:

Environmental triggers might be either preventable or inescapable. Different approaches are used for each.

If you're prepared to take additional precautions, you can avoid a lot of environmental triggers. Simply said, we often run into triggering circumstances because we're too proud to acknowledge our fragility. Avoiding environmental stimuli, however, does not indicate weakness.

Battle Advice 1: Steer clear of conflict

Jocko Willink, a former Navy SEAL captain and master in Brazilian Ju Jitsu, is about as difficult a tough person as you can find. But he offers straightforward guidance in hazardous circumstances: "Avoid confrontation if feasible."

Second, turn your gaze away. If you can, turn your head away or leave the area altogether. Third, celebrate your achievement—you have eliminated an environmental trigger!

We'll add a fourth to this: inform your ally. Speak to your friends if you can avoid the trigger easily or if you are having trouble. Tell them about the triggers in your surroundings. When you have allies, you have people who will support you in both success and failure.

2. Physical Reactions

How can the urge for porn be caused by our physical state? How can we prevent this? HALT stands for hungry and weary, which are bodily symptoms. You will be better able to combat porn if you improve your physical condition.

Why can't you do this? Discover your physical triggers and try to stay away from them. Physical triggers, like environmental stimuli, may often be avoided.

Because they are too exhausted and uninspired to accomplish anything else, a lot of individuals are lured to watch porn. After a hard day, some people find themselves inclined to rest and decompress by watching porn. Consider your physical state at the time of the trigger as well as the events that lead to it. Query these things:

- Having a healthy diet? Do you eat too much or not enough?
- Have you had enough water to drink?
- How about excessive caffeine intake?
- Do you frequently work out? Do you overwork out?

You may optimize your physical condition to prevent physical triggers by doing an accurate evaluation of your physical state. Make a war plan that gets you in the best possible physical shape to take on porn.

Numerous physical stimuli cannot be prevented. We all experience hunger, fatigue, and stress. Understanding your bodily state is crucial because it influences the best approach to dealing with your triggers. Do you feel jittery and irritated after drinking too much coffee? Reading a book may not be the best course of action in this situation. After a long day at work, are you exhausted and worn out? Exercise may not be beneficial in this situation.

Redirecting the trigger should be done from a position of strength rather than weakness.

Strategies for Redirecting Physical Triggers:

You may take action to reroute the physical trigger after you have a precise evaluation of it.

3. Find healthy alternatives to pornographic entertainment.

Consume some nutritious foods, such as raw fruit, veggies, or nuts. Sip on some water or tea without caffeine. To unwind, read a book or watch a (non-triggering!) television program.

Take a stroll.

Jump jacks or push-ups are good exercises.

Redirecting physical triggers may be accomplished by communicating with your allies. You need a supporter. Faced with physical triggers, a text or phone call may be a tremendous source of strength.

Recognize your limitations

Your physical resources are constrained. Sun Tzu once stated, "You can't make your vanguard stronger without making your rear-guard weaker."

To put it another way, your ability to combat porn may be diminished if you are working too hard in other aspects of your life. Take it easy on yourself. Prioritize your physical resources and make a plan to combat porn.

3. Emotional Reactions

Tom was a single guy in his late 30s who battled with porn and masturbation despite making every attempt to quit, according to counselor David Powlison.

Powlison finally questioned him over his most recent problem.

On Friday evenings, I'm worn out and alone, Tom added. I feel terrible for myself when I consider my single friends out on dates and my married friends with their spouses. I get upset with God because I feel like I should have a wife and I don't. By nine o'clock, I give in to the overpowering urge to commit a sexual transgression (David Powlison, Sexual Addiction, pp. 11-12). Take note of the feelings Tom mentions: rage, loneliness, and self-pity. These serve as emotional porn triggers. Emotions may be either good or bad. Environmental and physical causes might cause them, or they can be wholly unreasonable. Even professionals struggle to agree on how to define and classify emotions due to their complexity. You don't have to be a psychologist to understand your emotional triggers and to know who you are. Think back to the last time you were triggered and how you felt. How were you feeling?

Anger is one feeling that many people, including Tom, report being triggered by. Anger often drives people to engage in several damaging acts. There are many levels and types of anger as well; it might be fury, resentment, or even annoyance. Some circumstances may be upsetting at times. Be furious, but do not sin, Psalm 4:4 reads; "Search your heart on your bed and be calm."

In other words, you could have suffered injustice. Even yet, it is still wrong to sin. The psalmist advises you to "examine your heart and remain calm" rather than retaliating in fury. You may discover the sources of your rage, the sins you need to repent of, and the expectations you need to let go of by exploring your heart.

Because human rage does not result in God's righteousness, James 1:20 explains.

Sadness: Sadness and related feelings are often triggered. Depressive emotions such as feelings of loss, disappointment, loneliness, and others often act as triggers. Tom's rage was joined with regret and self-pity in his tale. Many different "downer" moods have the potential to lead to inappropriate porn behavior.

Many of the psalms struggle with grief. Waiting for the Lord "in the depths of affliction" is how Psalm 130 depicts it.

When faced with anxiety or uncertainty, porn might appear like an old and comfortable companion. Maybe you're having problems in your new career or your relationships. Since pornography temporarily offers the appearance of control, many people find that feeling vulnerable or out of control is a big trigger.

Anyone who is faced with scary situations can find great solace in Psalm 34. When I sought the Lord, he responded and rescued me from all of my worries (34:4).

Oh, taste and see that the Lord is good, and do not be drawn away by the seduction of iniquity! The one who seeks shelter in him is blessed. (34:8).

Joy: Other emotions than "downer" moods may also act as triggers for porn. Porn may result from emotions like

happiness, assurance, or control,
especially if you let your defenses down.

In my personal life, I find that I'm least
inclined to seek responsibility at the
periods when I feel the best about myself.
I think I don't need it. Pride precedes
disaster, and a haughty mind precedes a
fall, according to Proverbs 16:18.

Perhaps you're feeling pleased with
yourself for beating porn—great! Gratify
that. Happiness, though, might lead to
irresponsibility or disregard for the
methods that brought you success in the
past.

Wrestling porn

Only when a person decides to quit
seeing and fantasizing about porn can
recovery start.
A user has to be aware that internet porn
has the potential to lead to severe social,
mental, and physical health issues to be
motivated to attempt to quit using it. It
may potentially lead to a criminal record.
See How to identify a porn issue.
Take the glass out of the wound is a
saying at The Reward Foundation.
Everyone is aware that while a glass
fragment is still harming the body, a
wound cannot start to heal. So
eliminating the stressor of frequent
exposure to online porn allows the brain
to reset. It may then recover and
resensitize to regular arousal levels.
Start now

Start by deciding to give it up. You may use the tried-and-true precommitment strategy outlined in this study. It involves voluntarily limiting access to temptations and is effective with impulsive people. Set a one-day deadline for yourself. The goal is to begin identifying our own body's signals and improving our ability to react to them. Take note of the times of day that you tend to view porn. What does it feel like to be compelled to watch it? This is the mental tug-of-war sensation. To prevent the unpleasantness of having them absent, there is a need to experience a rush of pleasure neurochemicals. It conflicts with the need to demonstrate our self-control. This craving is a sign that the brain's dopamine or opioid levels are low. Arousal brought on by adrenaline triggers the stress response, urging us to "do something NOW!" But we have the power to resist such cravings, particularly if we prepare a plan in advance and are aware of when we are most vulnerable.

Being able to take a little break to consider things through before acting begins to weaken the neural pathway and stop the habit. It is a useful activity to attempt to break any bad habits we may have. It fosters self-control. One of the most crucial life skills for long-term success is that. It's just as significant as skill or intellect. Find out how others handled it after trying it. The anguish of restraint or the pain of regret must be chosen by each of us.

Screen Fast for one day

This may be used to determine a person's level of dependence on social networking, gaming, and porn.

Here is an extract from N. Postman and A. Postman's book Amusing Ourselves to Death: Public Discourse in the Age of Show Business. (Introduction).

"One professor utilizes the book in tandem with a 'e-media fast' experiment. Each pupil is required to abstain from using electronic devices for 24 hours. She informed me that 90% of the students shrug when she announces the assignment because they see it as being unimportant. However, "they start to whine and complain" when they discover all the things they have to give up for a whole day, including their mobile phone, computer, Internet, TV, and vehicle radio. They can still read books, however. Even though they will be sleeping for around eight of the twenty-four hours, she realizes that it will be a difficult day. She claims that they must start again if they break the fast—for example, if they need to answer the phone or merely check their email. The lecturer exclaims, "The papers I receive back are wonderful."

Abstaining

They are usually severe and have names like "The Worst Day of My Life" or "The Best Experience I Ever Had." They'll write, "I believed I was going to die." "I wanted to switch on the TV, but I thought, my God, I'd have to start over again," the speaker said. Every kid has a different area where they are weak—for some, it's TV, for others, their mobile phone, the internet, or their PDA. They take time to do things they haven't done in years despite how much they detest refraining from things or how difficult it is to hear the phone ring and not answer it.

To see their pal, they stroll down the street. They converse for a long time. One said, "I thought of doing things I had never dreamt of doing." They are altered by the encounter. Some people have such an impact that they decide to fast on their own, once a month. The classics I cover in that course—from Plato and Aristotle to the present—are what my former students remember when they write or phone to say hello years later.

The standing test

The son of the author of this book, which is in its twentieth edition, claims that his father's inquiries apply to all media and technology. What happens to us when we are tempted by them and then fall in love with them? Do they cage us or release us? Do they strengthen or weaken democracy? Do they increase or decrease the accountability of our leaders? Are our systems more or less transparent? Do they help us become better consumers or citizens? Are the sacrifices worthwhile? What tactics can we come up with to preserve control if they're not worth it but we still can't stop ourselves from embracing the next new thing because that's simply how we're wired? Dignity? Meaning?" See our news article to see how some sixth form students at an Edinburgh school fared through our 24-hour screen fast.

Use of pornography as a habit

To determine whether someone is habitually consuming online pornography, do this.

It is advisable to take this one-day elimination test for online pornography if you or someone you know wishes to. If you are successful, you may want to consider making the elimination last longer. It may be very simple to stop doing something for 24 hours, but it takes a week or three weeks to seemingly how obsessive a behavior has become.

The reboot might start practically immediately. Rebooters most often relapse during the first hour, the first day, and the first week because they are unable to resist the impulse to watch more. If you have been exposed to porn for a long period, it will take some time to break the habit. Rebooting is not a simple operation. If you do find it simple, simply express gratitude. Most people find it difficult. But being prepared means being prepared. It is very helpful to be aware of the emotional or physical symptoms that other rebooters have experienced on their road to recovery.

Cutting down versus giving up

Most obsessive behaviors don't respond well to harm reduction tactics like just reducing back. Finding a solution to quit watching pornography is no different. It may be much too simple to obtain a quick injection of feel-good hormones from our smartphone or tablet when we are agitated and have the want to "do something NOW!" Most individuals find that just cutting less on porn doesn't work since it only makes the habit last longer.

Too readily can the established routes be rekindled. To develop new, healthier pathways and avoid being sucked back in, it may take months or even years in some obstinate instances. Additionally, it may take multiple trial-and-error iterations to maintain the longer-term behavior of deterring ourselves from viewing porn. So consider these:

Stop consuming online porn.

Learn how to avoid porn on the internet 12 step, Programs like SMART recovery and mutual assistance may all be helpful.

Learn how the brain's reward system works. Abstinence is made simpler by realizing that this urge is a result of a dysregulated brain state.

Recognize the indications and triggers that cause your addiction to flare up. Learn how to prevent them.

Step 2: Train your mind

Most abstainers get something from psychological assistance. This might come from therapists who are professionals or from friends and family. This is where oxytocin levels in the brain may be increased through love in the form of hugs, cuddling, friendship, trust, and bonding. The numerous beneficial properties of oxytocin that serve to regulate the flow of electricity and neurochemicals include:

doespamine and cortisol (stress and depression) are offset (cravings)

decreases the withdrawal symptoms

enhances connections and feelings of security

reduces anxiety, dread, and concern sensations

Mindfulness
Regular, deep mental relaxation is one of the finest methods to develop resistance to life's pressures and strains. The term "Mindfulness" refers to one variant that is now quite popular. It entails briefly and non-judgmentally focusing our attention on whatever is on our minds or in our hearts. Instead than attempting to ignore or repress our anxious thoughts,
The majority of conflicts may be easily avoided by just paying attention to your surroundings. Recognizing you can win without fighting is not a sign of weakness. If a battle-tested martial arts master can experience this, then it is unquestionably true for those attempting to avoid porn. Do you have situational awareness? Are there any triggering locations you can stay away from to guarantee your continuous success in the war against porn? Are you prepared to do this even if it could mean losing out on some fun things? Try this if you're not sure. Then go back to what you were doing just before your most recent pornographic binge. Was there a way you may have prevented it?
Many individuals discover that even simply being alone themselves with a computer might be a trigger. Could this be prevented? Can you arrange plans in advance to keep yourself occupied with friends on the weekends and at other times when you may be alone? I once borrowed a friend's laptop from him for a while so I could avoid this trigger. A other young guy I know removed the door to

his bedroom to avoid the environmental trigger of being alone himself.

Even if you don't go to these lengths, you can utilize parental controls on your TV, Covenant Eyes filtering on your gadgets, and Screen Accountability.

Second battle tip: Take off the trigger Jesus asserts in Matthew 5:29–30 that it is preferable to amputate a hand or remove an eye than to fall into sin. In other words, if you're not ready to give up a little comfort or pleasure to avoid environmental triggers, you won't succeed.

But what about the environmental triggers that cannot be avoided? Perhaps it's a pop-up advertisement you weren't expecting or a billboard on a busy road. Sam Black provides a straightforward three-step solution in The Porn Circuit: warn, avoid, and confirm. To begin with, become aware of the environmental trigger. Recognize it for what it is and comprehend it

create time to address them, we let them into our minds and observe them without attempting to dismiss, fix, or even harshly evaluate them.

A potent mix of encouraging methods may be useful. Most increase oxytocin levels in us.

Cognitive behavioral therapy and mindfulness are effective together (CBT). While CBT targets the conscious, logical level to alter unfavorable thinking and perceptual patterns, mindfulness meditation targets the subconscious, nonverbal level that is deeper.

By encouraging insightful questions, motivational interviewing (MI) is effective in supporting adolescent drug users in their efforts to stop using drugs.
Stress-reduction program using mindfulness
We are not our thoughts. They are dynamic and subject to change. They do not have to control us; we can control them. They often develop into thought patterns, but if we are aware of them, we may alter them if they are not giving us happiness. Because they alter the kind of neurochemicals our brains create, thoughts can modify the structure of the brain over time and with enough repetition. We may become more cognizant of these underlying emotional drives and how they affect our emotions and feelings by practicing mindfulness. We have the power to regain it.
According to the findings of a Harvard Medical School research, where participants engaged in daily mindfulness activities for an average of 27 minutes, Amygdala's grey matter (nerve cells) reduced on MRI images (anxiety) Hippocampus has more grey matter, which improves memory and learning. produced psychological advantages that last all day Reported stress reductions recordings of free meditation
No cost meditation
Utilize our free deep breathing workouts to unwind and retrain your brain. Your body can heal if you stop the synthesis of stress neurochemicals. The power will assist your mind generate fresh concepts and insightful thoughts.

This first one will transport you to a sunny beach and is little under three minutes long. It immediately lifts one's spirits.
You may relax your muscles by using this second one. Although it just takes approximately 22.37 minutes, it may seem like 5.
In this third exercise, the goal is to unwind the mind without physically moving so that you may perform it in public or on the train. Duration: 18.13 minutes.
The fourth one lasts 16.15 minutes and takes you on a fantastical cloud-based journey. very soothing
Our last meditation, which helps you visualize goals for your life, lasts slightly over eight minutes.
When should profound relaxation occur? The optimum times to practice deep relaxation are early in the morning or late in the day. To avoid the digestive process interfering with your relaxation, leave at least an hour after eating or do it before meals. While it is often easiest to do it sitting up straight on a chair, some individuals prefer to do it while laying down. The only danger at that point is that you could nod off. Staying aware will allow you to deliberately let go of your anxious thoughts. You maintain control, therefore it's not hypnosis.
Step 3: Acquire important life skills
Some individuals need more of the "go get it" neurochemical, dopamine, to experience the same amount of drive and pleasure as someone who does not have that altered gene state. This is known as an in-born deficit or genetic

predisposition. A tiny portion of such persons are more susceptible to addiction than others. However, there are often two primary reasons why individuals engage in compulsive behavior or become addicted.

Why do people get addicted?

Like everyone else, they first seek pleasure and have fun, but little indulgences may quickly turn into regular routines. We are all susceptible to being seduced by the promise of "fun," even if it leads to missed deadlines, discomfort, hangovers, missed meetings, and broken promises. Over time, societal pressure and advertising may push us to binge on pleasures, which may physically alter our reward system in the brain and make cravings more difficult to suppress. Fear of missing out, or FOMO, is only a psychological trick played on us by society. Social media aids in the development of that specific brain worm. The second way addiction might emerge is from a subliminal desire to escape a difficult circumstance or task in daily life. It may occur as a result of a lack of life skills, such as the ability to deal with conflict, new experiences, meeting people, and family disputes. While seeking pleasure may initially ease tension or comfort pain, it is possible that in the long run it may cause more stress than the original issue. The effects of addiction make a person completely preoccupied with their demands and emotionally unavailable to others. As their stress levels rise, they begin to lose control of their lives. Advertisers promoting energizing pursuits like porn, booze, gambling, junk food, and gaming, to mention a few, profit from our propensity to look for enjoyment while ignoring unpleasant feelings or demanding circumstances.

Depression prevention

This may be changed, which lowers the likelihood of developing addictions and depressive disorders. Often, stopping the addictive behavior alone is insufficient. The individual will remain vulnerable and unable to handle criticism or confrontation since the trigger reaction to stress will still be there. There are several accounts of individuals who succeed in quitting drinking or using drugs and get a job, only to fall apart at the first sight of conflict and subsequently relapse. There are also inspiring tales of young people who quit up porn and get the bravery and fortitude to deal with challenging circumstances. Some people mention acquiring "superpowers."

Learning life skills to expand and grow one's life and make it more fascinating and rewarding helps people in recovery succeed and prevent relapse. It entails obtaining their motivation and enjoyment from more beneficial sources, particularly from face-to-face interactions, and letting go of feelings of guilt, shame, and unlovedness.

Numerous distinct life skills are proven to be beneficial, including:

coping mechanisms to improve bodily wellbeing

how to prepare and consume frequent, wholesome meals

obtaining enough restorative sleep—eight hours per night for adults, nine hours for kids and teenagers—is important.

Physical activity, particularly time spent in nature

Exercises for calming the mind, such as mindfulness or just allowing your thoughts to wander

Pilates, Tai Chi, and yoga

Life skills that increase self-assurance

Untrained minds are incapable of anything. Developing a new ability gradually helps boost confidence. It requires time. A mind that has been expanded cannot return to its original state. Nobody can take away from us a taught talent. We can endure in shifting situations more if we have greater talents. These abilities lessen the strain of a hectic lifestyle.

Control your thoughts, pessimism, and desires about becoming sexual

Home organization techniques include regular cleaning and shopping schedules as well as keeping vital documents, invoices, and receipts organized.

Learn how to submit a job application and be well-prepared for interviews.

Financial capability: developing a budget and, if at all feasible, a savings plan

www.ingramcontent.com/pod-product-compliance
Lightning Source LLC
Chambersburg PA
CBHW070228260726
48658CB00006BA/2224